5 ON 5 EATING CHALLENGE

10 Day Kick-off Meal Plan Included!

I0441459

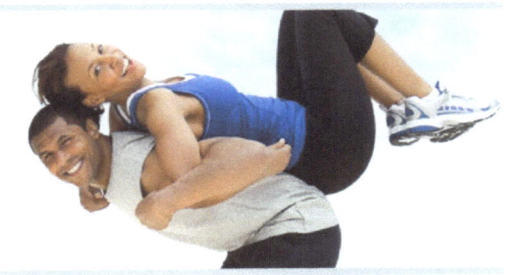

5 ON 5

THE MOST DOABLE WELLNESS
PLAN ON THE PLANET

Len Garrison
TrainwithLen.com

5 ON 5 is dedicated to the people, and teams of people, who have the desire to improve their quality of life, live longer and seek to leave a wellness legacy.

Foreward by Lori Woodward, RD

Other Books by Len

Stop And Think
5 ON 5!
Monday Mojo: 52 Ambition Instillations
The Chiseled Challenge for Men

Please visit TrainwithLen.com for updates on new materials.
"Your potential is my passion."

Part 1:
- What is this plan?
- What exactly do I do?
- Your 2 new favorite words: categories & portions

Part 2:
- Your 5 Categories!

Part 3:
- Your Eating & Shopping Chart

Part 4:
- Your 5 ON 5 Eating Challenge
- What to Eat When for 10 Days!

Part 5:
- Congrats on the Courage!
- Strike Management
- Add Your Own 5 Categories
- The Program of Life
- The Last Word

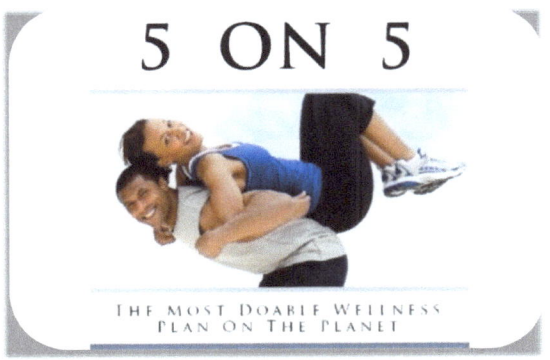

Foreward:

This book provides a great example of how we all should eat to maximize our nutritional health.   Readers of 5 On 5 will learn the most basic, yet useful information about eating for health. This book clearly describes the importance of meal planning, using the major macronutrients in our diet, and how these macronutrients play such an important role in our health and well-being.

Len has provided the key tools to help the reader understand how to create the most beneficial meal plan to increase metabolism, energy levels and blood glucose stabilization. With the information provided in this book, the reader will walk away with an increase in energy level, metabolism, and overall healthier lifestyle. The 5 on 5 book will give the reader a greater knowledge of the impact that nutrition has on our health, as well as the tools to create a successful personalized nutrition and exercise program.

I would recommend this book to anyone who not only desires a healthier long-term lifestyle, but to those who want to educate themselves on basic nutrition principles.

Yours in Health,
Lori Woodward, Registered Dietitian & Nutritionist

Part 1:

Live Your Life by Design | Create Your Own Upgrade

WHAT IS IT?

> The 5 ON 5 is a 10 week challenge designed with a holistic approach that will help develop new, healthy lifestyle habits! It is applicable to everyone at any level.

> This book is the **eating portion of the challenge only**. This book will challenge you to a 10 day kickoff plan, followed by a 5 week challenge (if you should choose to do so). For those who do not want another exercise routine, or have that area good-to-go, and simply want a strategy to incorporate healthier eating habits, this is your challenge! This is the 5 ON 5 eating challenge! Focus on your 10 days first. Your 11th day will be a free day, then decide if you want to rock out 5 weeks! You totally got this...

> For the entire challenge, with real live results from challenge finishers, please visit the TrainwithLen.com.

What Do I Do For The 1st 10 Days & the 5 Week Challenge?

Goal #1: Consume **ONLY** from these 5 categories for 10 days:
1. Water (coffee & tea ok- no artificial sweeteners)
2. Fruits
3. Veggies
4. Lean Proteins
5. Whole Grains

If you would like a deeper challenge, try this alongside the above goal:
- Eat 5 times per day for your 5 days.
  - You must eat 5 small meals per day for your 5 days. Nothing more, nothing less.

- You combine a fat, a carb and a protein for every meal.
- Since your body was meant to be fed not starved, eating this way boosts your metabolism for optimal fat burn, as well as fuel for your workout.
- The goal will be to get at least 3 servings of veggies and 2 servings of fruit per day. Timed eating will be your best bet. Your outlook just got busier!
- Try this: listen to your body and feed it when it's hungry. Make sure you eat something small every 3-4 hours, that combines a carb, protein and fat, and eat your larger meals only when you feel your stomach growl.

Goal #2: To score a 100!

- You must keep a food journal. Yup, you have to record everything that goes into your mouth for 10 days. It's the only way to know what you're made of ☺.
- Give yourself a score of up to 10 points per day for your 10 days. Keep your score in your food journal.
- Each of the 5 categories will be worth 2 points per day. Every day you will give yourself 2 points for eating / drinking from each of the 5 categories. If you miss eating one or more of the categories for that day, you will not earn those 2 points for that category.
- For example, if you eat fruits (2 points), veggies (2 points) and drink water (2 points), but do not eat any lean proteins (-2) or whole grains (-2), you will end up with a score of 6 points for that day. Don't worry, your category chart will help you know what foods are authorized.
- Each day you will score yourself with either a 2, 4, 6, 8 or 10.
- **After you rock your 10 days**, go for the same challenge 5 days a week for 5 weeks. Same scoring, up to 10 points per day, potential of 50 points per week, and a total of 250 point for your 5 weeks! Those other 2 days a week are your "off" days, take them if you like.

Goal #3: Finish! Don't give up. Even if day 3-4 are a total flop, kick it back in gear! Your 1st goal is to focus on your 1st 10 days.

Part 2:

5 ON 5 Eating Challenge | 10 Day Kick-Off

Congrats on accepting the 5 ON 5 challenge! It will be exciting and challenging at the same time! Why take on a challenge if it doesn't include both of those?

One of the best ways to accomplish your goal is to create your plan. Your plan is created by your own preparation. *Your preparation determines your destination*. For accountability, take some friends thru this with you! Get your team at work, your family, your school or your church involved. Make it a fun, interactive and competitive challenge! Maybe a prize at the end...

Having said that, it's time to write out what your week will look like for the upcoming week. Complete your list concerning how you will be active and what you will eat. Let's look at it...

Plan the work & work the plan!

Eat from only these 5 categories 5 days a week:
1. Water
2. Fruits
3. Veggies
4. Lean proteins
5. Whole grains

Here are the 2 most important words for your eating habits:
1. **Categories**
2. **Portions**

A portion is the size of your clinched fist. Keep it to **one portion per meal** per category. As much as you can, try to include a protein, a fat and a carb with each meal. This way you will promote an overall balanced intake and keep your energy high. Side note, if there is one word that sums up life, it's

balance. Eating this way by itself will increase your metabolism, which will kick in your natural fat burning mechanisms.

All food is made up of calories, and calories are separated into 3 distinct categories: carbohydrates, proteins and fats. If you are a calorie counter, there are approximately 9 calories per gram of fat, and 4 calories per gram of protein and carb, and you can figure it out from there. With this program, we are not concerned with calories, only categories. **Make your calories count vs. counting your calories**. The goal is to eat 5 small meals instead of the traditional 1-3 larger meals. Consider it grazing all day. Your body was meant to be fed, not starved. **As you fuel your body with the right foods more frequently, it will burn more rapidly**. Thus, coupled with being active, you will not give any excess calories a chance to hang around (literally). When you skip meals your body goes into survival, storage mode which will work against you. You need your body to constantly burn. The trick is to eat enough for this to take place without caloric overload. Fat is stored and accumulated when there is an excess of calories that your body can't use for energy. The way to achieve this is to focus on eating smaller meals more frequently and from the right sources. This way you only eat for what your body can burn and store for nutrient value. Anything more, or less, results in fat build up. Whether you eat too much, or not enough, it shows up the same way. Plan your intake with a well-rounded approach (no pun intended) and get into all 5 categories per day for the healthiest benefit. For example, grapes are authorized, but if you only eat grapes all day your diet will not be holistic, nor will your insulin level. The same applies to chicken or low fat cheese sticks. A whole and complete plate would look like: salmon (protein & healthy fats) with grilled asparagus (carbs); eggs (protein & healthy fats), whole grain toast and an apple (carbs); grilled chicken (protein) with baby spinach (carbs) topped with olive oil (fats)...

Try to remember the 70 – 30 rule. This means that you are *never* stuffed and you are *never* starving. 100% is all you can eat, stuffed, wheel me out of this feeding troth buffet. 0% is that you haven't eaten all day, your stomach is growling begging for substance, and you could "eat a horse." However, if you stay between 70% and 30% full, your metabolism is at its highest peak performance and burning fat for fuel.

100%----------------70%-------------------------30%------------------0%

Make your own eating plan from the category chart listed below. Pick and choose your favorites, or decide to eat the same thing 3-4 days in a row. I usually grill meat and veggies Sunday night and eat on it for the following few days in wraps, salads, sandwiches, etc.

The goal of the 5 ON 5 (you can get the entire book for complete info) is establishing healthier lifestyle habits. We are talking long term, not a temporary fix. With this program, we are concerned with categories, not calories. **This way**, you have the categories (or boundaries) to start from, and now you have the creativity to create in your kitchen! *It causes you to think and prepare and do,* which are the keys to creating a habit. The categories act as guidelines. You prepare healthy meals with healthy ingredients for you and your family, not from some other diet fad. You need to be able to have room for creative thinking, meal preparation and time spent cooking for the long term effects to be produced.

Serve up heart-healthy foods. Try to get **5 servings per day of fruits & veggies**, 3 veggies and 2 fruits are good. It could be 3 servings of veggies (the size of your fist) and 2 servings of fruit (one apple and one banana), or anyway you chose. It helps to lower LDL ("bad") cholesterol and adds antioxidants to your intake.

Strategy for the weekends: get in your head an idea of what you will eat from your 5 categories for upcoming week. Make a shopping list and get what you will need by Sunday night. This way you will not have the tendency to **eat haphazardly** throughout the week. Planned eating is the best way to keep your nutrition goals. Just remember: *categories and portions*. Stay within your boundaries and practice your portions. If it doesn't fit into the 5 categories it doesn't fit into your shopping cart!

You can make more food equal fewer pounds. You can actually get away with eating more food if you eat from the right categories. It's not about high and low, it's about good and bad.

For example:

- You could eat ½ of a dry bagel worth 200 calories **–OR–** you eat 2 wheat waffles with 2 teaspoons of raw honey and berries for 200 calories.

- You could eat a 9 ounce muffin worth 720 calories **–OR-** you can eat 1 pineapple, ½ of a cantaloupe, ½ kiwi fruit, ½ papaya, grapes, 2 pears and 2 whole wheat rolls for the same amount – 720 calories.
- You could eat 1 chicken nugget for 80 calories **–OR-** you could eat a cup and a half of vegetable soup for the same 80 calories.
- You could eat 2 slices of cheese pizza for 900 calories **–OR-** you could eat 1 slice of cheese pizza, ½ cup of minestrone, and side salad with vinaigrette for 600 calories.
- You could eat 1 fat free cookie for 60 calories **–OR-** you can eat one entire cantaloupe for 60 calories.
- You could have a vodka drink and a cup of chips for 740 calories – **OR-** you could have 1 cup of consommé, 5 oz of scallops, sides of asparagus and red cabbage, tossed salad, 1 wheat roll, strawberries and 1 cup of red wine for 740 calories.
- You could have one oversized chocolate chunk cookie for 640 calories **–OR-** you can have 2 frozen yogurt cones, a large plate of fruit, 6 hard candies, and 8 pieces of dark chocolate for 640 calories.

So you see, eating from the right categories can create more food, which in turn equates to fewer pounds. It's truly a win win!

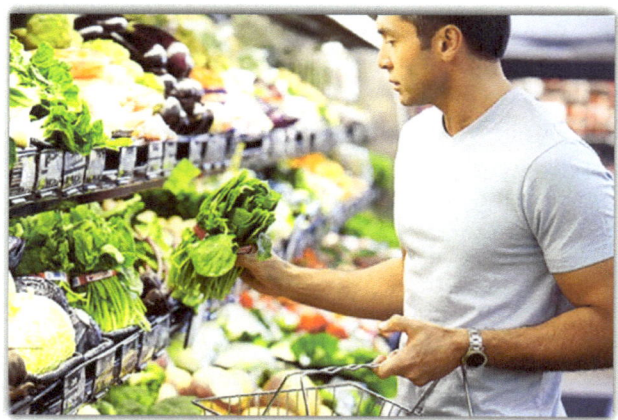

Part 3:

Your 5 Categories

1). WATER.
Water only? Limited amounts of coffee, tea and red wire are allowed on the 5 ON 5. Let me explain...

Coffee and tea are great until we put sugars, flavored syrups and saturated fats into them. On this plan there are **NO** false sweeteners, such as aspartame (NutraSweet & Equal), Splenda, saccharin (sweet & low). Stay away from words like "sugar substitute", "artificial sweetener", and "sugar free." Only two cups per day of coffee or tea. One coffee and one tea, or two cups of coffee and no tea, and so on. You can use 1 teaspoon of all natural honey, skim milk, 1 packet per cup of sugar-in-the-raw, Stevia, Agave sweetener, Truvia or cinnamon. 1-2 glasses of red wine are allowed. See, you knew this was going to be an awesome program! And **you must have** a glass of water *coupled* with your coffee, tea or red wine. The reason those 3 liquids are allowed is because most people love them, and in moderation they have many health benefits. Come on, you can do this for 10 days! Never have only **one** drink by your side. Practice taking one drink of water for every one drink of coffee, tea or red wine. Go double fisted. Be aware that the majority of your liquid intake must be water. The best rule for water intake is to divide your body weight in half, and that is how many ounces per day to shoot for. Water hydrates your body, fights off fatigue and free radicals. It prevents joint soreness, promotes organ health, muscle strength and brain function.

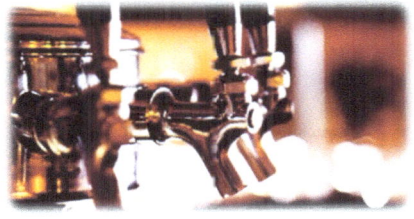

THE LIQUID INTAKE

Be mindful of your liquid intake. It's too easy to sabotage your diet by drinking excess sugars, salts, full fat dairy or alcohol. The two most obvious observations are soft drinks and too much alcohol consumption.

> "More Americans now drink sugar-sweetened sodas, sport drinks and fruit drinks daily, and this increase in consumption has led to more diabetes and heart disease over the past decade, researchers reported at the American Heart Association's 50th Annual Conference on Cardiovascular Disease Epidemiology and Prevention."

ScienceDaily (Mar. 6, 2010)

An average person can save 15 pounds per year (especially dudes) simply by cutting soft drinks and sugary drinks out of their diet. Listen to some of these stats according to Weightloss.org:

- 21% of all sugar in the average American diet comes from soft drinks.
- Drinking 1 soft drink per day increases your risk of metabolic syndrome by 44% and increases the risk of childhood obesity by 60%.
- Drinking 2 soft drinks per day increases your risk of gout by 85%.

"Have you ever noticed that soft drinks sometimes leave you more thirsty? A 12 ounce can of coke has 50 grams of added sodium (salt), and the salty taste covered by the 40 grams of added sugar. This added salt in the soda may influence you to drink more compared to drinking water. Dietary salt is a major determinant of how much fluid we drink."

GreenliteMedicine.com / Greenlite Medicine on Wed, Mar 23, 2011

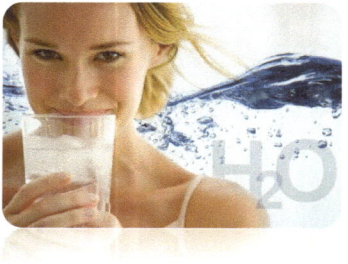

It's pretty obvious soft drinks will not get you where you want to go. The fact is, **to go up you have to recognize what you have to give up**. Keep reminding yourself that discipline equals freedom, and freedom is the energy for life. You overcome cravings with mind power. The battle field is always in the mind field first. If you are stuck on soft drinks, sweet tea or other sugar laden drinks, just begin with small switches. For example, always have water next to other drinks and alternate drinks, replace a coke with tea- ½ sweet and ½ unsweet with a lemon, or unsweet tea with fruit. Also try cucumber or coconut water. Begin these switches and practice **steady strategic progression**. Do not replace a soft drink with an "energy" drink. Seek out all natural liquids, 100% fruit juice, no added sugar, and please drink what comes from the earth not from a factory.

Here is the issue with alcohol: it naturally boosts cortisol, which is a fat storage hormone, and the higher the alcohol content the higher the calories, which do convert to sugars. Alcohol also slows down your metabolism. Ouch… And there is 7 calories per gram of alcohol. Knowledge is power. If you want to abide by a law for leanness, limit your alcohol to 1-2 drinks per day, and take some off days from drinking any.

> "Over time, excessive alcohol consumption can decrease insulin's effectiveness, resulting in high blood sugar levels. One study showed that 45% to 70% of people with alcoholic liver disease had either glucose intolerance or diabetes. Get the facts on how **alcohol** impacts nutrition, metabolism, diet and weight loss, blood **sugar**, vitamins and minerals."
> *Medicinenet.com*

As you are getting more natural foods in you, you are getting preservatives, sedatives, additives and chemically enhanced items out. That means your body is producing more natural chemicals to fight against fat and free radicals. Free radicals are atoms that damage red blood cells. They speed up the aging process, weaken the immune system and cause diseases. They get in you from eating fried foods, smoking, drinking too much, allowing too much fat to store, lack of exercise, and simply unclean eating. Stored fat cells hold onto harmful free radicals and muscle tone helps to thwart them off. Foods that are rich in antioxidants: red beans, blueberries, kidney beans, strawberries, blackberries, apples, plums, etc; combat those suckers.

Having said that, if you want to shoot for water only on your 5 days, go for it! You may want to do that if your goal is to completely detox your body of sugars, caffeine and alcohol.

How *do you* keep eating from only 5 categories? Just like most good things in life, it's simple in theory but harder in practice. Easier said than done, but then again who said it would be easy? Anything you do worthwhile, and that carries meaning, has to cost you something. I know you can completely do this! You just have to determine which one you **want** more. **Do you want your goals or your cravings?** You have to fortify in your mind that temporary sacrifice now equals feeling really good later. You may want that pie, but you want your goals more. I know you do! You want your accomplishment and success more than you want unclean foods. Literally picture that pulling into the drive thru means pulling out your bigger pants. Visualize those fries ending up as fat around your waist. You are eating your way to larger love handles. What you are eating is adipose tissue- or pure fat- that will hang around your waist. **Looseness in your diet equals looseness around your waist.** Your cravings will try to tempt you, lead you down the negative path. Think of all that follows us when we don't eat clean. It affects our moods, self-esteem, and our soul.

The more you stick to a goal and complete it, the more your soul is empowered.

The idea behind the 5 ON 5 eating plan is to put into our bodies what God made, not what a factory made. Moving to foods in their natural state is the goal. In sales training, they use the phrase "switch and get rich." The same applies here. Start with small switches. Switch your sweet tea for half & half, or unsweet with a lemon and an orange slice. Switch your hamburger to a turkey burger with a whole wheat bun, switch your fries for a side salad, switch to light beer, switch your muffin for a wheat waffle, switch your regular pizza for wheat flour, organic flatbread, organic sauce and veggies! You get the idea. Keep in mind that every bit counts and **small switches make the big difference**. Over the course of time, significant change will not occur without daily differences. It's the day in day out small choices that make the biggest difference!

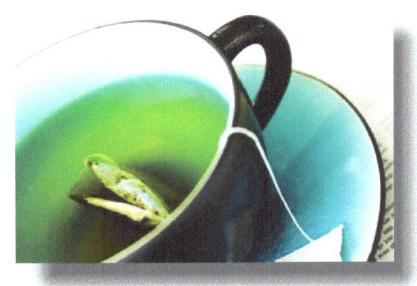

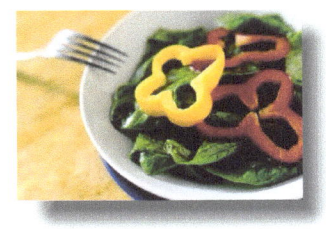

2). FRUIT (any fruit works, you can't get more natural than that)

Blueberries
Raspberries
Apples
Peaches
Clementine's

Pineapple
Oranges /

Strawberries   Grapes / Bananas
Pears   Blackberries

3). VEGGIES (any raw veggie)

Spinach   Fresh mushrooms
Tomatoes   Carrots
Celery   Onions
Black beans   Cucumber
Water chestnuts   Pickles
Scallions
Tomatoes
Romaine lettuce   Sweet potatoes

Broccoli   Bell peppers

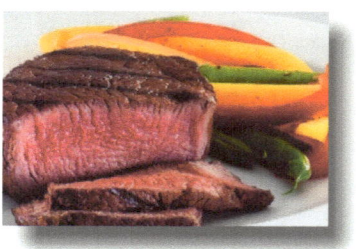

OILS/DRESSINGS
Extra virgin olive oil
        All natural Cooking spray
Olive oil or balsamic vinaigrette
        Italian vinaigrette
Fruit based dressings
        Herb based dressings
Coconut oil

4). <mark>LEAN PROTEINS</mark>

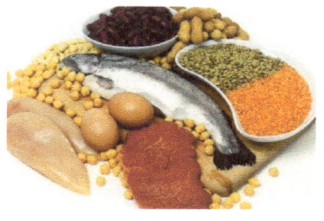

Skinless chicken breasts
New York choice lean sirloin steak
Low-fat sliced chicken
Turkey deli meat
Eye of round beef steak

Ground turkey
Turkey burgers
Turkey bacon
Lean ground beef
Low fat dairy
All natural peanut butter
Low sodium ham
Soy

FISH

Canned tuna (packed in water)
Mahi Mahi
Salmon filet

Flounder
Trout
Haddock
Seafood

DAIRY (low fat)

Grated low-fat Parmesan cheese
Low-fat cheese slices
Shredded cheeses
String cheese
Low fat sour cream

Skim milk
Fresh or organic eggs
Greek yogurt
Low fat yogurt
Soy

BEANS, NUTS & SEEDS

Almonds	Brazil nuts	Black bears
Cashews	Chestnuts	Kidney beans
Peanuts	Pecans	Garbanzo
Pistachios	Walnuts	White beans
Chia	Flax	Pinto beans
Hemp	Poppy	Lentils
Sesame	Sunflower	Split peas

5). ==WHOLE GRAINS== (Complex carbs)

Old-fashioned oatmeal / Steel cut
Whole grain flour
Low-fat whole-wheat frozen waffles
Whole-wheat:

- English muffins
- Pita bread
- Bread & buns
- Spaghetti

Brown rice
Quinoa, buckwheat, amaranth
Whole grain, long or wild rice

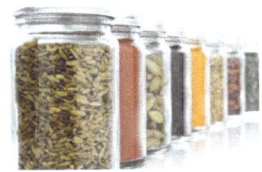

SPICES

Cinnamon
Pepper
Sea Salt
Paprika

Chili powder
Ginger
Cilantro (love it)
Oregano

Garlic powder	Basil
Cloves of fresh garlic	Dill week
Cumin	Parsley

TOPPINGS/CONDIMENTS

Fresh lime juice (be mindful of added sugar)	Fresh salsa
Light teriyaki marinade	Stevia or Truvia
Almonds/slivered almonds	Lemon or lime juice
All natural peanut butter	Mixed nuts
Green enchilada sauce	Low sodium ketchup
Spicy mustard	All natural Agave sweetener
Low sodium Soy sauce	

<mark>Lighter = leaner. Eat right, eat light, eat healthy.</mark>
O M E G A ' S :

You can make your weekly menu from this list or simply use it for ideas. For **dinner it's a good idea to go with lean & green.** Stick to a lean protein and green colorful veggies. For a leaner approach, taper off starches throughout the day, and consume your wheat's and other grains for breakfast and lunch.

The comparison between your on days and your off days will be apparent to your system. And over the course of the 10 weeks you will begin to feel the vast and better difference of being "on" much more than begin "off." Your taste buds will begin to feel what they were intended to feel and your system will crave clean eating. Your body will recognize the healthy sources you are feeding it. Your brain will be clearer, your complexion will look smoother, your blood sugar will stabilize and your energy will increase! This way you have them side by side, eating clean as well as eating unclean. You will be able to feel the vast difference and therefore prove to yourself eating clean wins.

I know you will find good results and new eating habits will form. You know it's happening when healthy food tastes better than it used to and your body begins to reject the unclean things.

It's all about a progression, even if it's only little by little. As a matter of fact that is the healthiest way to go. **Consistency** and a focus on the overall process, not how much you weigh today, is the goal. Remember that it's what we do and how we think *on the journey* that counts, not simply reaching a destination. We want to put practices in motion that will cause us to live healthier and do healthier things. When you put unfair expectations on yourself, you immediately put your health goals in jeopardy. So take unnecessary pressure off, it's not about going buck-wild insanity or quick fixes.

Consistency and focus on the overall process is the goal, not how much you weigh today.

Progress can be fast or slow, either way it's progress. Day in and day out focus on your categories, stay active and get your points. As you wrap your brain around what to eat and when to eat it, you are instilling a life habit. So keep it up! Every bit counts. The result will be carryover and lifestyle changes – forever!

On this plan, the other 2 days feel free to eat what you wish. They are yours. If you know you can have that stack of pancakes in two days, it will help you hold of eating anything uncategorized today. I enjoy my free days. That doesn't mean I go hog wild on them, but it does mean I allow myself to eat a variety of things. It's a healthy thing to let your taste buds go and eat whatever you want 1-2 days a week. And when the next week comes it is different, get back on it! That practice is ok. Why would I say that? Because the program is about a balanced life. **If we create that life balance now, realistic intake and expenditure, we are more apt to stay on healthier habits on weeks 20, 30 and beyond...**

Because numbers can get in your psyche in a negative way and detour your motivation, **I would not encourage scale watching. Rather, focus on what you can see, feel and fit into!** Recognize the power of process, and watch as your body fat (more vital than body weight) is reduced. It wasn't put on overnight and it will not go off overnight. Put a pair of jean you have wanted to fit back into on the door. Leave them there as a reminder. Hang that dress up in the bathroom. *Instead of weighing yourself, view yourself in the mirror.* Take weekly pictures instead of the traditional weekly weigh in. If you do choose to weigh in, understand realistically a healthy weight drop is typically 1-2 pounds per week for females and 2-3 for males. I also am not a fan of the BMI. If you must go with a number system go with your body fat % and your measurements using body tape.

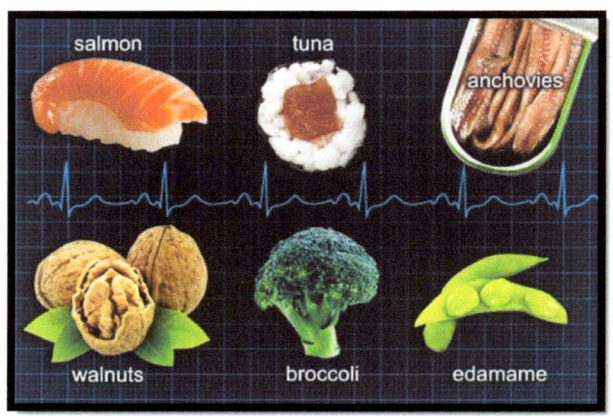

5 ON 5 Example Meals

YOU GOT THIS...

Breakfast	Lunch	Dinner	Healthy Snacks
Egg whites or 1 whole egg	Turkey in a spinach wrap, extra veggies. Hold the mayo, switch to spicy mustard or vinaigrette	Grilled chicken 2 sides of veggies	Protein shake (w/out false sweeteners)
Wheat toast or whole grain waffles, 1 teaspoon of raw honey.	Whole wheat pasta with grilled chicken (one portion), one avocado	6 oz fillet steak, grilled OR 2 "skinny" burgers Served with 1 Tbsp tangy tomato salsa 4 oz baked	All natural peanut butter with apple slices or 3 celery stalks

		potato with 1 tsp low fat sour cream	
1 whole wheat bagel or English muffin with fruit	Cold chicken from yesterday, sliced, with light mayo Leaf salad with vinaigrette	Salmon with 2 sides of veggies	Low fat cheese with whole grain crackers
100% whole grain cereals with skim milk	4 oz tuna packed in spring water, served with salad, capers, and olives	Turkey chili	1 cup of low fat cottage cheese
Oatmeal with fruit 	Grilled chicken burrito (fresh veggies and salsa, whole wheat or spinach wraps)	1 portion New York choice lean sirloin steak, grilled 1 portion steamed asparagus 1 small yam or sweet potato	1 cup fruit
Egg white and Avocado Sandwich (use 1 slice whole-wheat bread)	Salad with chicken 1 portion raspberries Glass of water	Chicken Whole Wheat Pasta Primavera Glass of water	Carrot sticks and low fat ranch
Omelet (Authorized ingredients)	Tuna Salad Apple	Grilled Mahi Mahi 2 veggies for sides	Greek Yogurt
Banana pancakes (whole wheat flour, 2 tps honey or all natural agave sweetener)	Tuna Melt (use 1 tbsp low-fat cheese and whole-wheat bread)	Sushi made with brown rice, seaweed salad	Cup of warm nonfat milk with 1/2 tsp honey 1 apple

| | 1 portion almonds | |

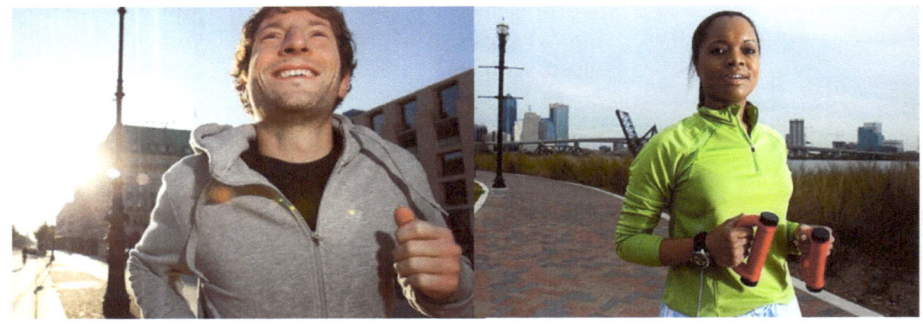

Part 4:

10 Day 5 ON 5 Eating Challenge

Each day is based on an average of 1700 calories. For men, you may want to add additional protein to take your calories up to around 2000-2200. For example, use two salmon filets, two chicken breasts, extra turkey, protein shake, 2 eggs, etc. This way you also get extra protein and fiber so you can keep your muscles full.

You can mix and match a little bit according to your likes, but keep it clean, category driven and watch your portions. The important thing is to write out exactly what you eat on these 10 days, good and bad! There is nothing like the discipline of writing out what you ate, it gives a visual of your real intake.

Your goal is to score a 100! See page 5 for instructions.

- Eating 5 small meals per day boosts your metabolism and fat burning mechanisms. (You don't have eat 5 meals to get points, they come from watching categories, but it is a good goal to shoot for). Think of it as 3 meals and 2 snacks. Each time you eat do your best to consume a protein, a carb and a fat.

- Don't skip meals and do not skip breakfast.
- Consider it as grazing all day. For example, a grizzly bear eats only one big meal every few days, sleeps too much and has an enormous amount of body fat. An Elk is one of the leanest and strongest animals, and they simply graze on vegetation all day and get exercise. Be an Elk.
- A portion is the size of your fist.
- Always be double fisted. Not with brew, but with water. Always have water with any other liquid intake, and alternate drinks.
- Take your body weight and cut it in half, that is how many ounces of water you need per day.
- Do your best to get a healthy portion of carbs, proteins and fats for every meal.
- Shortcuts never pay off in the long run.
- Fat lasts longer than flavor.
- Run through roadblocks.
- Well begun is half done.
- Plan the work and work the plan!

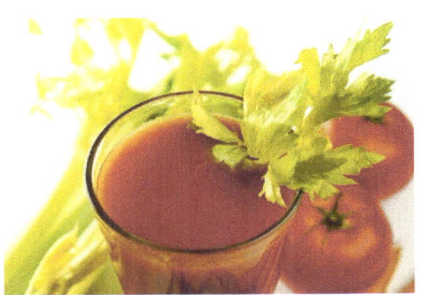

Monday Day 1

Planned   Actual

Breakfast	
2 scrambled eggs & 1 piece of whole grain toast / Ezekiel bread ½ or whole banana	
Snack	
Greek Yogurt	

Lunch	
Grilled chicken and veggies inside a spinach tortilla 1 apple	
Snack	
2 scoops of all natural peanut butter and a banana or protein shake	
Dinner	
Whole Wheat Pasta with salmon or shrimp: size of your fist. Salad with 2 Tbsp olive oil/vinegar dressing. Blueberries for dessert	

Score:

Tuesday Day 2

Planned   Actual

Breakfast	
2 pieces of turkey bacon and 1 egg Handful of blueberries or strawberries	
Snack	
1 piece string cheese and black beans	
Lunch	
Leftover Whole Wheat Pasta with tuna on top 1 apple	
Snack	
25 almonds	
Dinner	
Rotisserie Chicken with wild rice 2 cups of broccoli 2 cups of snow peas	

Score:

Wednesday Day 3

Planned	Actual
Breakfast	
All natural oatmeal with blueberries and 2 teaspoons of all natural peanut butter	
Snack	
Protein bar or shake (**grams of sugar are not to exceed grams of protein**)	
Lunch	
Leftover Chicken with wild rice 1 apple	
Snack	
Greek yogurt	
Dinner	
Grilled chicken (olive oil & spices) with baby spinach 2 cups of broccoli	
Snack	
Pineapple slices	

Score:

Thursday Day 4

Planned	Actual
Breakfast	
Loaded Vegetable Omelet 1 banana	
Snack	
Beef jerky (low sodium)	
Lunch	
Eat Out (keep it clean: no fried foods, beer or	

excess sugars)	
Snack	
1 piece of fruit & edamame	
Dinner	
Steamed or grilled Snapper with asparagus Salad with 2 Tbsp olive oil/vinegar dressing	

Score:

Notes: (What's working & what needs tweaking?)

Friday Day 5

Planned	**Actual**
Breakfast	
3 Scrambled Eggs (2 egg whites, 1 whole egg) 1 orange	
Snack	
Handful of Almonds and an apple	
Lunch	
Turkey Wrap Side salad balsamic vinaigrette	
Snack	
1 protein bar	
Dinner	
Grilled or baked salmon 1 sweet potato and broccoli	

Score:

Saturday Day 6

Planned	Actual
Breakfast	
2 whole wheat waffles, no syrup, add blueberries and/or peanut butter 1 banana	
Snack	
Protein drink or 2 scoops of peanut butter and a banana	
Lunch	
Grilled chicken salad 1 apple	
Snack	
15 baby carrots 2 Tbsp of hummus 1 piece of string cheese	
Dinner	
Grilled Cilantro-Lime Chicken Salad with 2 Tbsp olive oil/vinegar dressing 1 sweet potato	

Score:

Sunday Day 7

Planned	Actual
Breakfast	
Egg white omelet with veggies 1 serving of Greek yogurt	
Snack	
Cucumber slices with hummus	
Lunch	
Black Bean burger or grilled chicken on whole wheat bun	

side salad with olive oil or balsamic vingarette	
Snack	
1 piece of string cheese and a handful of grapes	
Dinner	
Turkey chili	

Score:

Yeah baby! You made it, you're 1st week! Congrats. Now reward yourself. Take a free meal, dessert or just go buy some new jeans!

Monday Day 8

Planned   **Actual**

Planned	Actual
Breakfast	
3 scrambled eggs 1 banana	
Snack	
Low fat cheese with whole grain crackers	
Lunch	
Grilled chicken and veggies inside a spinach tortilla 1 apple	
Snack	
2 scoops of all natural peanut butter and a banana or protein shake	
Dinner	
Whole wheat pasta with salmon or shrimp: size of your fist Salad with 2 Tbsp olive oil/vinegar dressing Blueberries for dessert	

Score:

How does your body feel? Taste buds changing? In tune with your tummy?

Tuesday Day 9

Planned	Actual
Breakfast	
Lean low sodium ham and 2 eggs Handful of blueberries or strawberries	
Snack	
25 almonds	
Lunch	
Leftover Whole Wheat Pasta with Vegetables 1 apple	
Snack	
Cucumber slices and hummus	
Dinner	
New York choice lean sirloin steak (portion size of you fist) 2 cups of broccoli 2 cups of snow peas	

Score:

Wednesday Day 10

Planned	Actual
Breakfast	
Oatmeal with blueberries and 2 teaspoons of all natural peanut butter	
Snack	
Mix1 or greek yogurt	
Lunch	
Cold chicken from yesterday, sliced, with light mayo Leaf salad with vinaigrette	
Snack	
25 almonds	
Dinner	
Chicken Spinach Parm 2 cups of broccoli	
Snack	
Pineapple slices	

Nice! I knew you had this.

Part 5:

CONGRATULATIONS

Congratulations on finishing! I knew you would find the courage and discipline!

Regardless if you scored a 100 or a 50, you have established new lifestyle habits. Realize it or not you have set positive patterns in motion. The score is simply a number, an extra motive, a measure to get some of these healthier habits in action. Since they are now part of you, the discipline will

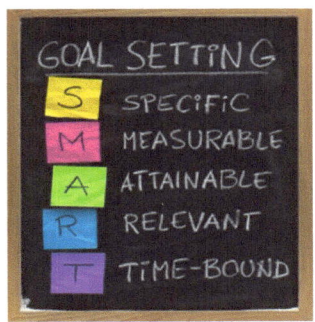

naturally come out. **Reject old, unclean, unhealthy habits. They are no longer an acceptable part of your life.** That doesn't mean you can't have your free days, but it does mean that 80% of your week will be clean & healthy!

Keep setting your goals, planning the work and working the plan, setting up your seasons and ultimately living by design. Go thru the 5 ON 5 again and take someone thru it with you! One thing is for sure, what you get going gets going. The longer you practice this discipline the more it will develop into second hand nature, which will produce the longer living and thriving you!

SYSTEMATIC & PROGRAMMATIC

Each 10 days or 5 weeks that you compete in this challenge, you will find it a worthwhile season and experience several growth points. Take those growth points and keep adding them to your new life. Continue to create new and improved life cycles. Remember you have to be your own best trainer, so continually keep yourself accountable and challenged.

Set up your year!

A neat idea that has worked for me and the programs I run is to outline my year in semesters. I encourage you to do the same ☺. Write out what you will do for the spring, summer and fall semesters. The important thing is to develop your system. Draft what it will look like and put it on display. Display it on your frig, your home office, social media, etc. Below are 2 examples of ones I have created for our program at work. You can draft your layout for yourself, your family, your career, etc.

Think of it in terms of **"steady strategic progression."** You are leading your life to stages of achievement and progress.

Everything functions better on a program, and you maximize your long term efforts by making it systematic. Keep it up and keep moving, allow your program to develop, and in the meantime it is *becoming* systematic. A natural flow is what you want, that will be the goal and it will happen.

"The first and greatest victory is over self."
~Plato

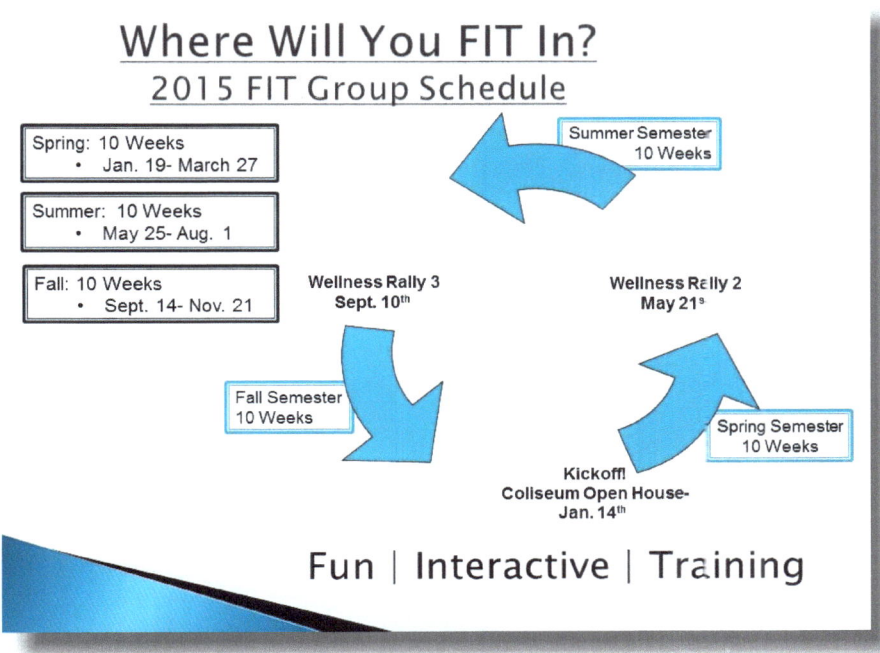

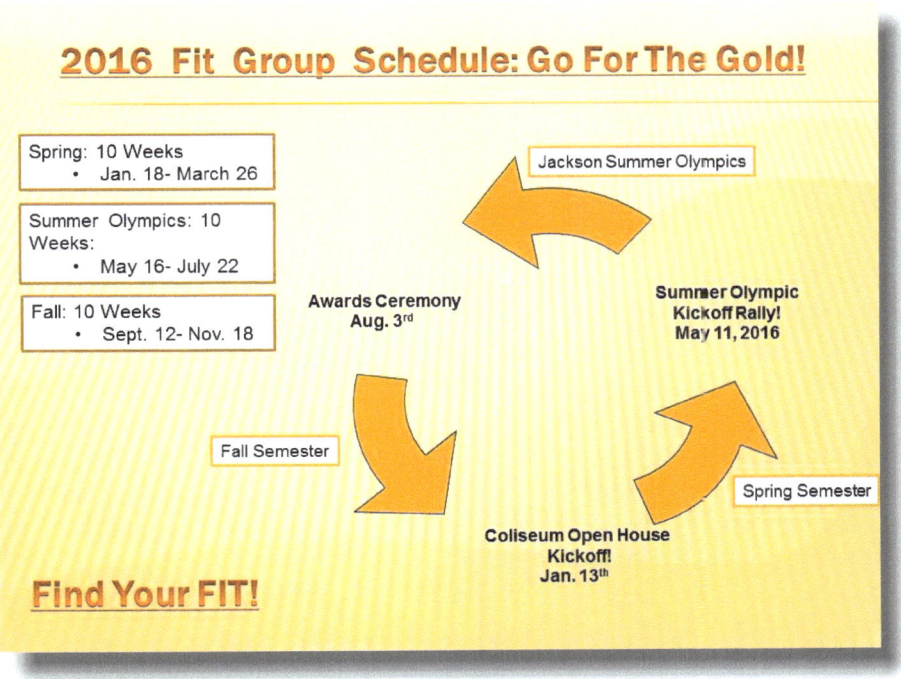

CATEGORIES & PORTIONS

These two words have been hammered home and need to remain part of your constant vocabulary. These two disciplines will- above all else- allow you the transformation you want. Remember categories, not calories. A portion size is the size of your clenched fist.

Discipline brings freedom and freedom is the energy in life.

Feeling the pinch now means you will be able to pinch less later!

STRIKE MANAEGMENT

One thing is true about opportunity, you don't wait until the iron is hot to strike, you keep striking your own iron until it gets hot. It doesn't knock either, you have to go find it. Now is your time to create opportunity for yourself.

Nike has a philosophy on "strike management" that I like. They are talking about running and their running shoes. The idea is to use "designed features to guide the foot from heel to toe." They explain how to strike the pavement and release off your toes in the correct way. They have different shoes for different problem areas. Their selling points are cushioning of the midsole, arch support, curbs knee pain, gets rid of excessive pronation, and to help with all phases of the foot strike. Similarly, the 5 ON 5 is going to assist you with strike management for your life! **It's an awesome thing when you learn how and when to strike for mental empowerment, nutrition, exercise, holistic health and programmatic living.** That's why it's vital to set up your year. Some semesters you will need to strike harder on your nutrition, some semesters exercise, some brain power, some emotional stability, some family connectedness, etc. The encouragement here is to take Nike's example of strike management and apply it to your life! Pay attention to your current life status and your overall wants in life, and begin striking today with good management.

ADD YOUR OWN 5 CATEGORY TO YOUR NEXT SEMESTER

Another thing that is great about this program is that you can create your own challenge according to your level and interest. Once you have completed your first 5 ON 5, you can add different levels to your next 5 ON 5. **Customize your training and make it relative** to where you are and what you are going for. For example, alongside the parameters of eating from only 5 categories:

- Eat 5 small meals per day 5 days a week
- Eat 5 servings of veggies per day
- Exercise 5 days a week
- Take 10 group fitness classes during your 5 weeks
- Hire a trainer for 10 sessions
- Run a 5k 5 days a week
- Complete 5 5k race events (or other events) during your 10 weeks
- Swim or bike 5 days a week
- Do your 1st 5k, marathon or triathlon at the end of your 10 weeks
- Set a progression workout where you have a goal of benching x amount
- Feed your mind 5 times per day 5 days a week
- Learn 10 new yoga poses in 10 weeks
- Receive your certification at the end of your 10 weeks
- Make your active level 30 or 40 minutes 5 days a week
- If you are a dancer, make your activity dancing 3-5 days a week

What else?

THE PROGRAM OF LIFE

"Intelligence is your ability to adapt to change."
Albert Einstein

Life has cycles and seasons. The ones who make the most of it are working on where they are and where they are going. The seasoned individuals take advantage of the time and wisdom they do have- always.

My encouragement is to take a panoramic view of your own life's program- past, present and future. Looking at the past you can see patterns that do not need to be repeated and habits that need correcting. Recognizing where you *are* allows you to soak in the moment (and the emotion of the moment), and understand how you got here. *Visioneering* steers your ship and keeps you focused and motivated on your next phase. All 3 are important and key parts to make up a whole, a whole life that is.

As you are working on your 5 weeks and your yearly format, you are really working on your lifelong program. What you do now directly affects your tomorrow. It's common in business to develop a 1 year plan, 3 year, 5 year and so on. **Why not do the same with the business of life?** Strike a deal with yourself about your health. It's your life, create your program.

Talking in terms of authoring your own life's program, there is a really good read entitled *What Is Your Life's Work?* by Bill Jensen. This book is about capturing what really matters to people. Bill has interviewed people from all walks of life and all across the globe to find out what they feel really matters and what does not. He asked questions like, "What's the single most important insight about work and life that you want to pass on to your kids? Or to anyone you truly care about?" Some of the captions that caught my eye are:
- "Be a respectful rebel."
- "Honey, there are no shortcuts."
- "Speak up if you don't agree."
- "The only way to get what you want is to see that you already have what you need."
- "Be real, put yourself out there. Your work diary is a tool for others self-discovery."

- "Our mind, body and spirit can be their own unique healers when we let them."
- "Entitlement is not an option. Earn your income."
- "You will do magical things in your life. You need to believe that."
- "Always choose family."

Bill puts a life cycle into 5 categories:
1. Finding yourself
2. Finding the lessons to be learned, the questions to be asked
3. Finding the choices that really matter
4. Finding the courage to choose
5. Finding joy, serenity and fulfillment

I love it. The only thing I would add to that is leaving a legacy. I am a father of 3 beautiful and talented kids. You better believe my mot vation for all I do is leading by example now and leaving behind a legacy for them to follow.

Live life by design not by default

Take-A-Way Tip:

Be an ACE by sticking with vitamins A, C & E daily. These are a great combo and when combined together, with regular intake. they produce:
- A higher level of antioxidants that prevents cancer and cardiovascular disease.
- Protection against the harmful effects of pollution, carcinogens, protects against infection, and enhances immunity.
- A greater enhancement of our eyes, organs and skin.
- A reduction in the potential harmful buildup around the arteries.
- A greater fight to degeneration.
- A reduced the risk of Alzheimer's disease and osteoporosis.

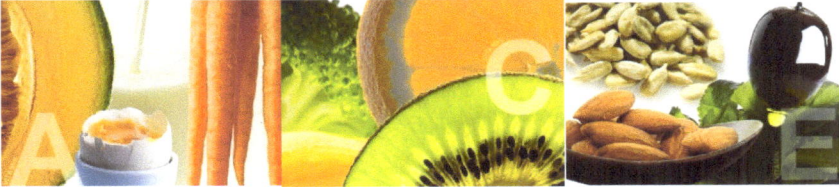

"Make your potential your passion.

Then make the potential of others your passion."

Life by design,

Len Garrison

TrainwithLen.com

www.ingramcontent.com/pod-product-compliance
Lightning Source LLC
Chambersburg PA
CBHW050757290526
45792CB00008B/2222